Table of Contents

INTRODUCTION 3

CHAPTER ONE 5

    Bariatric Surgery 5

    Types 5

    Reasons for Bariatric Surgery 6

    Who it's for 6

    Risks 8

    Preparation 9

    What you can expect 10

    Types of bariatric surgery 11

    After bariatric surgery 13

    Results 14

    When weight-loss surgery doesn't work 15

CHAPTER TWO 16

    Gastric Bypass Diet 16

    Diet details 17

    Liquids 19

    Pureed foods 20

    Soft foods 20

    Solid foods 21

    A new healthy diet 23

Results 25
Risks 25
Recipes 26
CONCLUSION 84

INTRODUCTION

Before undergoing gastric bypass surgery, you must first qualify for the surgery and understand the risks and benefits involved. Adults eligible for this surgery are typically more than 100 pounds overweight or have a body mass index (BMI) over 35.

You may also be eligible if your BMI is between 30 and 35, your health is at risk due to your weight, and making lifestyle changes hasn't led to weight loss, according to the American Society for Metabolic and Bariatric Surgery (ASMBS).

To be a viable candidate, you should also be ready to re-learn your dietary habits. New dietary habits can help ensure the surgery has positive and lifelong effects.

Before your surgery, you need to make plans for a special diet to follow both pre- and post-surgery.

The pre-surgery diet is geared toward reducing the amount of fat in and around your liver. This reduces the risk of complications during the surgery.

After the surgery, your doctor will tailor the general diet guidelines for you. The post-surgery diet usually consists of several weekly phases. It helps you recover, meet the needs of your now smaller stomach, and gain healthier eating habits.

Losing weight before surgery helps reduce the amount of fat in and around your liver and abdomen. This may allow you to have a laparoscopy rather than open surgery. Laparoscopic surgery is less invasive, requires much less recovery time, and is easier on your body. Losing weight prior to surgery not only keeps you safer during the procedure, but it also helps train you for a new way of eating.

Your exact eating plan and pre-op weight loss goal will be determined by your healthcare provider and likely with the help of a registered dietitian.

Your eating plan may begin as soon as you're cleared for the procedure. If sufficient weight loss doesn't occur, the procedure may be postponed or canceled. For this reason, you should start the diet plan as soon as you can.

CHAPTER ONE

Bariatric Surgery

Gastric bypass and other weight-loss surgeries — known collectively as bariatric surgery — involve making changes to your digestive system to help you lose weight. Bariatric surgery is done when diet and exercise haven't worked or when you have serious health problems because of your weight. Some procedures limit how much you can eat. Other procedures work by reducing the body's ability to absorb nutrients. Some procedures do both.

While bariatric surgery can offer many benefits, all forms of weight-loss surgery are major procedures that can pose serious risks and side effects. Also, you must make permanent healthy changes to your diet and get regular exercise to help ensure the long-term success of bariatric surgery.

Types

1. Biliopancreatic diversion with duodenal switch (BPD/DS)
2. Gastric bypass (Roux-en-Y)
3. Sleeve gastrectomy

Reasons for Bariatric Surgery

Bariatric surgery is done to help you lose excess weight and reduce your risk of potentially life-threatening weight-related health problems, including:

- Heart disease and stroke
- High blood pressure
- Nonalcoholic fatty liver disease (NAFLD) or nonalcoholic steatohepatitis (NASH)
- Sleep apnea
- Type 2 diabetes

Bariatric surgery is typically done only after you've tried to lose weight by improving your diet and exercise habits.

Who it's for

In general, bariatric surgery could be an option for you if:

- Your body mass index (BMI) is 40 or higher (extreme obesity).

- Your BMI is 35 to 39.9 (obesity), and you have a serious weight-related health problem, such as type 2 diabetes, high blood pressure or severe sleep apnea. In some cases, you may qualify for certain types of weight-loss surgery if your BMI is 30 to 34 and you have serious weight-related health problems.

Bariatric surgery isn't for everyone who is severely overweight. You may need to meet certain medical guidelines to qualify for weight-loss surgery. You likely will have an extensive screening process to see if you qualify. You must also be willing to make permanent changes to lead a healthier lifestyle.

You may be required to participate in long-term follow-up plans that include monitoring your nutrition, your lifestyle and behavior, and your medical conditions.

And keep in mind that bariatric surgery is expensive. Check with your health insurance plan or your regional Medicare or Medicaid office to find out if your policy covers such surgery.

Risks

As with any major procedure, bariatric surgery poses potential health risks, both in the short term and long term.

Risks associated with the surgical procedure can include:
- Excessive bleeding
- Infection
- Adverse reactions to anesthesia
- Blood clots
- Lung or breathing problems
- Leaks in your gastrointestinal system
- Death (rare)

Longer term risks and complications of weight-loss surgery vary depending on the type of surgery. They can include:
- Bowel obstruction
- Dumping syndrome, which leads to diarrhea, flushing, lightheadedness, nausea or vomiting
- Gallstones
- Hernias

- Low blood sugar (hypoglycemia)
- Malnutrition
- Ulcers
- Vomiting
- Acid reflux
- The need for a second, or revision, surgery or procedure
- Death (rare)

Preparation

If you qualify for bariatric surgery, your health care team gives you instructions on how to prepare for your specific type of surgery. You may need to have various lab tests and exams before surgery. You may have restrictions on eating and drinking and which medications you can take. You may be required to start a physical activity program and to stop any tobacco use.

You may also need to prepare by planning ahead for your recovery after surgery. For instance, arrange for help at home if you think you'll need it.

What you can expect

Bariatric surgery is done in the hospital using general anesthesia. This means you're unconscious during the procedure.

The specifics of your surgery depend on your individual situation, the type of weight-loss surgery you have, and the hospital's or doctor's practices. Some weight-loss surgeries are done with traditional large, or open, incisions in your abdomen.

Today, most types of bariatric surgery are performed laparoscopically. A laparoscope is a small, tubular instrument with a camera attached. The laparoscope is inserted through small incisions in the abdomen. The tiny camera on the tip of the laparoscope allows the surgeon to see and operate inside your abdomen without making the traditional large incisions. Laparoscopic surgery can make your recovery faster and shorter, but it's not suitable for everyone.

Surgery usually takes several hours. After surgery, you awaken in a recovery room, where medical staff monitors you for any complications. Depending on your procedure, you may need to stay a few days in the hospital.

Types of bariatric surgery

Each type of bariatric surgery has pros and cons. Be sure to talk to your doctor about them. Here's a look at common types of bariatric surgery:

- Roux-en-Y (roo-en-wy) gastric bypass. This procedure is the most common method of gastric bypass. This surgery is typically not reversible. It works by decreasing the amount of food you can eat at one sitting and reducing absorption of nutrients. The surgeon cuts across the top of your stomach, sealing it off from the rest of your stomach. The resulting pouch is about the size of a walnut and can hold only about an ounce of food. Normally, your stomach can hold about 3 pints of food. Then, the surgeon cuts the small intestine and sews part of it directly onto the pouch. Food then goes into this small pouch of stomach and then directly into the small intestine sewn to it. Food bypasses most of your stomach and the first section of your small intestine, and instead enters directly into the middle part of your small intestine.

- Sleeve gastrectomy. With sleeve gastrectomy, about 80% of the stomach is removed, leaving a long, tube-like pouch. This smaller stomach can't hold as much food. It also produces less of the appetite-regulating hormone ghrelin, which may lessen your desire to eat. Advantages to this procedure include significant weight loss and no rerouting of the intestines. Sleeve gastrectomy also requires a shorter hospital stay than most other procedures.
- Biliopancreatic diversion with duodenal switch. This is a two-part surgery in which the first step involves performing a procedure similar to a sleeve gastrectomy. The second surgery involves connecting the end portion of the intestine to the duodenum near the

stomach (duodenal switch and biliopancreatic diversion), bypassing the majority of the intestine. This surgery both limits how much you can eat and reduces the absorption of nutrients. While it is extremely effective, it has greater risk, including malnutrition and vitamin deficiencies. Which type of weight-loss surgery is best for you depends on your specific situation. Your surgeon will take many factors into account, including body mass index, eating habits, other health issues, previous surgeries and the risks involved with each procedure.

After bariatric surgery

After weight-loss surgery, you generally won't be allowed to eat for one to two days so that your stomach and digestive system can heal. Then, you'll follow a specific diet for a few weeks. The diet begins with liquids only, then progresses to pureed, very soft foods, and eventually to regular foods. You may have many restrictions or limits on how much and what you can eat and drink.

You'll also have frequent medical checkups to monitor your health in the first several months after weight-loss surgery. You may need laboratory testing, blood work and various exams.

Results

Gastric bypass and other bariatric surgeries can provide long-term weight loss. The amount of weight you lose depends on your type of surgery and your change in lifestyle habits. It may be possible to lose half, or even more, of your excess weight within two years.

In addition to weight loss, gastric bypass surgery may improve or resolve conditions often related to being overweight, including:
- Heart disease
- High blood pressure
- Obstructive sleep apnea
- Type 2 diabetes

- Nonalcoholic fatty liver disease (NAFLD) or nonalcoholic steatohepatitis (NASH)
- Gastroesophageal reflux disease (GERD)
- Osteoarthritis (joint pain)

Gastric bypass surgery can also improve your ability to perform routine daily activities, which could help improve your quality of life.

When weight-loss surgery doesn't work

Gastric bypass and other weight-loss surgeries don't always work as well as you might have hoped. If a weight-loss procedure doesn't work well or stops working, you may not lose weight and you may develop serious health problems.

Keep all of your scheduled follow-up appointments after weight-loss surgery. If you notice that you are not losing weight or you develop complications, see your doctor immediately. Your weight loss can be monitored and factors potentially contributing to your lack of weight loss evaluated.

It's also possible to not lose enough weight or to regain weight after any type of weight-loss surgery, even if the procedure itself works correctly. This weight gain can happen if you do not follow the recommended lifestyle changes, such as getting regular physical activity and eating healthy foods.

CHAPTER TWO

Gastric Bypass Diet

A gastric bypass diet helps people who are recovering from sleeve gastrectomy and from gastric bypass surgery — also known as Roux-en-Y gastric bypass — to heal and to change their eating habits.

Your doctor or a registered dietitian will talk with you about the diet you'll need to follow after surgery, explaining what types of food and how much you can eat at each meal. Closely following your gastric bypass diet can help you lose weight safely.

Purpose

The gastric bypass diet is designed to:
- Allow your stomach to heal without being stretched by the food you eat
- Get you used to eating the smaller amounts of food that your smaller stomach can comfortably and safely digest
- Help you lose weight and avoid gaining weight
- Avoid side effects and complications from the surgery

Diet details

Diet recommendations after gastric bypass surgery vary depending on your individual situation. A gastric bypass diet typically follows a staged approach to help you ease back into eating solid foods. How quickly you move from one step to the next depends on how fast your body heals and adjusts to the change in eating patterns. You can usually start eating regular foods about three months after surgery.

At each stage of the gastric bypass diet, you must be careful to:

- Drink 64 ounces of fluid a day, to avoid dehydration.
- Sip liquids between meals, not with meals. Wait about 30 minutes after a meal to drink anything and avoid drinking 30 minutes before a meal.
- Eat and drink slowly, to avoid dumping syndrome — which occurs when foods and liquids enter your small intestine rapidly and in larger amounts than normal, causing

nausea, vomiting, dizziness, sweating and diarrhea.
- Eat lean, protein-rich foods daily.
- Choose foods and drinks that are low in fats and sugar.
- Avoid alcohol.
- Limit caffeine, which can cause dehydration.
- Take vitamin and mineral supplements daily as directed by your health provider.
- Chew foods thoroughly to a pureed consistency before swallowing, once you progress beyond liquids only.

Liquids

For the first day or so after surgery, you'll only be allowed to drink clear liquids. Once you're handling clear liquids, you can start having other liquids, such as:

- Broth
- Unsweetened juice
- Decaffeinated tea or coffee
- Milk (skim or 1 percent)
- Sugar-free gelatin or popsicles

Pureed foods

After about a week of tolerating liquids, you can begin to eat strained and pureed (mashed up) foods. The foods should have the consistency of a smooth paste or a thick liquid, without any solid pieces of food in the mixture.

You can eat three to six small meals a day. Each meal should consist of 4 to 6 tablespoons of food. Eat slowly — about 30 minutes for each meal.

Choose foods that will puree well, such as:
- Lean ground meat, poultry or fish
- Cottage cheese
- Soft scrambled eggs
- Cooked cereal
- Soft fruits and cooked vegetables
- Strained cream soups

Blend solid foods with a liquid, such as:
- Water
- Skim milk
- Juice with no sugar added
- Broth

Soft foods

After a few weeks of pureed foods, and with your doctor's OK, you can add soft foods to your diet. They should be small, tender and easily chewed pieces of food.

You can eat three to five small meals a day. Each meal should consist of one-third to one-half cup of food. Chew each bite until the food is pureed consistency before swallowing.

Soft foods include:
- Ground lean meat or poultry
- Flaked fish
- Eggs
- Cottage cheese
- Cooked or dried cereal
- Rice
- Canned or soft fresh fruit, without seeds or skin
- Cooked vegetables, without skin

Solid foods

After about eight weeks on the gastric bypass diet, you can gradually return to eating firmer foods. Start with eating three meals a day, with each meal consisting of 1 to 1-1/2 cups of food. It's important to stop eating before you feel completely full.

Depending on how you tolerate solid food, you may be able to vary the number of meals and amount of food at each meal. Talk to your dietitian about what's best for you.

Try new foods one at a time. Certain foods may cause pain, nausea or vomiting after gastric bypass surgery. Foods that can cause problems at this stage include:
- Breads
- Carbonated drinks
- Raw vegetables
- Cooked fibrous vegetables, such as celery, broccoli, corn or cabbage
- Tough meats or meats with gristle
- Red meat
- Fried foods
- Highly seasoned or spicy foods
- Nuts and seeds
- Popcorn

Over time, you might be able to try some of these foods again, with the guidance of your doctor.

A new healthy diet

Gastric bypass surgery reduces the size of your stomach and changes the way food enters your intestines. After surgery, it's important to get adequate nourishment while keeping your weight-loss goals on track. Your doctor is likely to recommend that you:

- Eat and drink slowly. To avoid dumping syndrome, take at least 30 minutes to eat your meals and 30 to 60 minutes to drink 1 cup of liquid. Wait 30 minutes before or after each meal to drink liquids.
- Keep meals small. Eat several small meals a day. You might start with six small meals a day, then move to four meals and finally, when following a regular diet, three meals a day. Each meal should include about a half-cup to 1 cup of food.
- Drink liquids between meals. To avoid dehydration, you'll need to drink at least 8 cups (1.9 liters) of fluids a day. But drinking too much liquid at or around mealtime can

leave you feeling overly full and prevent you from eating enough nutrient-rich food.
- Chew food thoroughly. The new opening that leads from your stomach into your small intestine is very narrow and can be blocked by larger pieces of food. Blockages prevent food from leaving your stomach and can cause vomiting, nausea and abdominal pain. Take small bites of food and chew them to a pureed consistency before swallowing.
- Focus on high-protein foods. Eat these foods before you eat other foods in your meal.
- Avoid foods that are high in fat and sugar. These foods travel quickly through your digestive system and cause dumping syndrome.
- Take recommended vitamin and mineral supplements.After surgery your body won't be able to absorb enough nutrients from your food. You'll likely need to take a multivitamin supplement every day for the rest of your life.

Results

The gastric bypass diet can help you recover from surgery and transition to a way of eating that is healthy and supports your weight-loss goals. Remember that if you return to unhealthy eating habits after weight-loss surgery, you may not lose all of your excess weight, or you may regain any weight that you do lose.

Risks

The greatest risks of the gastric bypass diet come from not following the diet properly. If you eat too much or eat food that you shouldn't, you could have complications. These include:

- Dumping syndrome. If too much food enters your small intestine quickly, you are likely to experience nausea, vomiting, dizziness, sweating and diarrhea. Eating too much or too fast, eating foods high in fat or sugar, and not chewing your food adequately can all cause nausea or vomiting after meals.
- Dehydration. Because you're not supposed to drink fluids with your meals, some people

become dehydrated. That's why you need to sip 64 ounces (1.9 liters) of water and other fluids throughout the day.
- Constipation. A lack of physical activity and of fiber or fluid in your diet can cause constipation.
- Blocked opening of your stomach pouch. Food can become lodged at the opening of your stomach pouch, even if you carefully follow the diet. Signs and symptoms of a blocked stomach opening include ongoing nausea, vomiting and abdominal pain. Call your doctor if you have these symptoms for more than two days.
- Weight gain or failure to lose weight. If you continue to gain weight or fail to lose weight on the gastric bypass diet, talk to your doctor or dietitian.

Recipes

Here are some recipes to try on after a gastric bypass surgery

Yogurt Breakfast Popsicles

INGREDIENTS

- 1 cup Greek yogurt, plain, non-fat
- ½ cup milk 1% or skim
- ½ cup regular or instant oats
- 1 cup mixed berries or chopped fruits

DIRECTIONS

1. Mix together the milk and yogurt.
2. Divide the mixture between your popsicle molds.
3. Place a few berries into each mold.
4. Divide the ½ cup oatmeal among each mold.
5. Place a wooden ice cream stick into each mold and place the popsicles into the freezer for at least 4 hours before eating.
6. To remove the popsicles, run the mound under a little hot water until they come loose.

Shrimp Ceviche

INGREDIENTS

- 1 pound medium raw shrimp

- 1 cup lime juice (approximately 5 fresh limes)
- 4 medium tomatoes (Roma or Italian), diced OR 8 ounces canned, diced tomatoes
- 1 small red onion, peeled, finely chopped (approximately ¾ cup chopped)
- 1 bunch cilantro, stemmed and finely chopped
- 2 serrano chili peppers, ribs and seeds removed, minced (optional)

Tip: For a mild option, try half of a medium green bell pepper.

DIRECTIONS

1. In a bowl, combine shrimp and lime juice.
2. Cover and marinate for about 10 to 15 minutes or until color changes to pink. Do not marinate too long, as the shrimp will "overcook" and toughen.
3. Add onions, tomatoes, chili peppers and cilantro.
4. Gently stir to combine.
5. Season with salt to taste.

6. Serve cold.

Chicken Caprese
INGREDIENTS
- 1 pound boneless, skinless chicken breasts
- 1 tablespoon olive oil
- 1 teaspoon dry Italian seasoning (or equal parts of garlic powder, dried oregano and dried basil)
- 4 thick (½-inch) slices ripe tomato
- 4 1-ounce slices fresh mozzarella cheese
- 3 tablespoons balsamic vinegar
- 2 tablespoons thinly sliced basil
- Pepper to taste

DIRECTIONS
1. Heat a grill or grill pan over medium high heat.
2. Drizzle 1 tablespoon of olive oil over chicken breasts and season to taste with and pepper.
3. Sprinkle Italian seasoning over the chicken.
4. Place the chicken on the grill and cook for 3 to 5 minutes per side, or until done. Cook

time will vary depending on the thickness of your chicken breasts.

5. When chicken is done, top with a slice of mozzarella cheese and cook for 1 more minute.
6. Remove from heat and place chicken breasts on a plate.
7. Top each breast with one slice of tomato, thinly sliced basil and pepper to taste.
8. Drizzle with balsamic vinegar or balsamic glaze and serve.

Black Bean and Corn Salad
INGREDIENTS
- 1 cup corn, whole kernel
- 2 cans (16-ounces each) black beans, rinsed and drained
- ¼ cup parsley, chopped fresh
- 2 tablespoon red onion, minced
- ¼ cup balsamic vinegar
- 2 tablespoon olive oil
- 1 teaspoon lemon juice

- 1 teaspoon garlic, minced
- 1 teaspoon honey or brown sugar
- Dash salt
- ¼ teaspoon ground black pepper

DIRECTIONS
1. Mix fresh corn, black beans, red onion and fresh parsley together in a large mixing bowl.
2. Whisk together balsamic vinegar, olive oil, lemon juice, garlic, honey, salt and pepper.
3. Pour over black beans and corn mixture.
4. Let the salad marinade for 30 minutes before serving.

Peanut Applesauce Chicken
INGREDIENTS
- 2½ pounds chicken pieces
- ¼ cup yellow mustard
- ⅛ cup Splenda brown sugar, unpacked
- ½ cup powdered peanuts
- Salt and pepper to taste
- 1 (15 ounce) jar applesauce, unsweetened

DIRECTIONS
1. Cook chicken in sauté pan.

2. Once nearing fully cooked, add applesauce, mustard, brown sugar and powdered peanuts.
3. Stir ingredients together.
4. Simmer over medium heat until an internal temperature of 165°F is reached.

Spicy Peanut Vegetarian Chili
INGREDIENTS
- 1 tablespoon peanut oil (or canola oil)
- 1 cup chopped onion
- 2 cloves garlic, minced
- 2 tablespoons chili powder
- 1 teaspoon chipotle chili pepper (optional)
- ¼ teaspoon dried oregano
- 1 can (16 ounce) black beans, drained and rinsed
- 1 can (16 ounce) white beans, drained and rinsed
- ⅔ cup powdered peanuts
- 1 can (28 ounce) diced tomato
- 1 can (15 ounce) tomato sauce
- 2 cups vegetable broth

DIRECTIONS
1. In a large Dutch oven, heat oil over medium high heat.
2. Add onion and garlic, sautéing 3 – 4 minutes or until tender.
3. Stir in chili powder, pepper, oregano and salt.
4. Sauté 2 minutes or until fragrant.
5. Add beans, corn, powdered peanuts, tomatoes, tomato sauce and broth.
6. Bring to a boil.
7. Reduce heat and simmer for about 30 minutes.

Note: This recipe may be cooked in slow cooker for 2 – 3 hours.

Peanut Butter and Jelly Pancakes
INGREDIENTS
- ½ cup low-fat cottage cheese
- ½ cup instant oatmeal
- 2 tablespoons powdered peanuts
- 4 large egg whites
- 1 cup frozen mixed berry blend

DIRECTIONS

1. Put Items in a blender in this order: cottage cheese, oatmeal, powdered peanuts and egg whites.
2. Turn on blender and blend until smooth like pancake batter.
3. Pour into a bowl and fold in berry fruit mix.
4. Use cooking spray in skillet. Makes 4 to 7 pancakes depending on size.

Peanut Powder Salad Dressing
INGREDIENTS
- 2 tablespoons powdered peanuts
- 1 tablespoon soy sauce, low sodium
- 1 tablespoon water
- ⅛ teaspoon garlic powder
- ¼ teaspoon ground pepper
- ¼ teaspoon Szechuan chili sauce
- 1 teaspoon Splenda brown sugar blend
- ⅛ teaspoon sesame oil

DIRECTIONS

Blend all ingredients well and serve. Refrigerate any remaining sauce.

Pumpkin-Ricotta Protein Pie

INGREDIENTS
- 2 cups 100% pure pumpkin puree, canned, without salt
- 2 eggs, large
- 1 cup milk, nonfat (skim milk)
- 1 cup ricotta cheese, part skim
- ⅓ cup Truvia for Baking or Splenda Sugar Blend
- 2 scoops 100% Unflavored Whey Protein Isolate (such as BiPro 1 scoop=~22 grams)
- ½ teaspoon salt
- 1 teaspoon cinnamon, ground
- 1 teaspoon nutmeg, ground
- 2 ounce package pecan halves

DIRECTIONS
1. Preheat oven to 350°F.
2. Spray 9-inch pie dish and 4 small ramekins with nonstick spray.

3. Blend ricotta cheese, eggs and ½ cup of milk until smooth, it should be liquid-like.
4. Add remaining ingredients and blend until smooth.
5. Pour liquid mixture into sprayed cooking dish, decorate with pecans on top.
6. Bake for 40 – 45 minutes or until middle is set and fairly solid. It should not jiggle when fully cooked. The sides and center should brown and grow up to double its size. If you experience over-browning on the top, reduce temperature to 325°F for the remainder of the cooking time.
7. Cool for 1 hour before cutting. This also allows for the pie expansion to settle.
8. Slice into 12 even pieces with a clean knife. Wipe the knife between each slice for a clean cut.

Tip: If you decide to use a crust (such as graham cracker, or regular pie pastry, you will need to adjust the nutrition information and calories upwards accordingly.

High-Protein Pumpkin Pie Oatmeal

INGREDIENTS
- ⅓ cup old fashioned oats (30 grams)
- ½ cup pumpkin, canned
- ⅛ teaspoon cinnamon
- Dash ground cloves
- Dash ground ginger
- 1 teaspoon Truvia baking blend
- ½ cup no salt added 1% cottage cheese

DIRECTIONS
1. Combine oats, pumpkin, spices, and sweetener in a microwave safe bowl.
2. Microwave on high for 90 seconds.
3. Stir in the cottage cheese.
4. Microwave on high for 60 seconds.
5. Let sit for a couple of minutes before eating.

Apple and Tuna Sandwiches Recipe

INGREDIENTS
- 1 can tuna, packed in water (6.5 ounces, drained)

- 1 apple
- ¼ cup yogurt, low-fat vanilla
- 1 teaspoon mustard
- ½ teaspoon honey
- 6 slices whole wheat bread
- 3 lettuces leaves

DIRECTIONS

1. Wash and peel the apple. Chop it into small pieces.
2. Drain the water from the can of tuna.
3. Put the tuna, apple, yogurt, mustard, and honey in a medium bowl. Stir well.
4. Spread ½ cup of the tuna mix onto each 3 slices of bread.
5. Top each sandwich with a washed lettuce leaf and a slice of bread.

Baked Chicken With Vegetables

INGREDIENTS

- 4 potatoes, sliced
- 6 carrots, sliced
- 1 large onion, quartered

- 1 chicken, raw, cut into pieces with skin removed
- ½ cup water
- 1 teaspoon thyme
- ¼ teaspoon pepper

DIRECTIONS
1. Preheat oven to 400 degrees.
2. Place potatoes, carrots and onions in a large roasting pan.
3. Put chicken pieces on top of the vegetables.
4. Mix water, thyme and pepper. Pour over chicken and vegetables.
5. Spoon juices over chicken once or twice during cooking.
6. Bake for one hour or more until browned and tender.

Silky Chocolate Soy Dessert Recipe
INGREDIENTS
- 1 envelope unflavored gelatin
- ¼ cup hot water

- 1 package (1.4 oz) sugar-free, fat-free chocolate fudge instant pudding
- 1 cup cold skim milk
- 16 ounces silken tofu
- ½ teaspoon vanilla extract
- 1 tablespoon cocoa powder (optional)
- ¼ teaspoon peppermint extract (optional)

DIRECTIONS

1. In a small bowl, mix the hot water and unflavored gelatin. Set aside and allow to firm.
2. In a medium-sized bowl, combine the cold skim milk and instant pudding mix.
3. Dice the tofu into ½- to 1-inch cubes and place in bowl with pudding mixture. Quickly whisk together to break up the soy cubes.
4. Add the vanilla extract and optional cocoa powder and peppermint extract.
5. Spoon the pudding and tofu mixture into a blender or food processor. Blend until smooth. You may need to blend for about 5

seconds and hand mix or shake the contents so that the motor does not stick.
6. Once the mixture has a smoothie-like texture, gradually add the gelatin until well combined and blend again.
7. Pour into a glass 8-inch dish, cover and place in refrigerator for at least 30 minutes to firm. The longer it sits, the firmer it will become.
8. Cut into eight portions and enjoy!

Pork and Black Bean Verde Stew Recipe
INGREDIENTS
- 2 teaspoons extra-virgin olive oil
- 1 pound pork loin or tenderloin, trimmed of visible fat and cut into 1" cubes
- 1¼ cup chopped onions
- 3 cloves garlic
- 2 canned chipotle peppers in adobo sauce, minced plus 1 teaspoon adobo sauce
- 1 teaspoon ground cumin
- 1 packet Goya Sazon with coriander & annatto (or similar seasoning packet)

- 1 can (14 ounces) no salt added chicken broth
- 1 can (14.5 ounces) no salt added diced tomatoes in juice
- 1 can (14.5 ounces) no salt added black beans, drained & rinsed
- 1 teaspoon crushed red pepper flakes (optional)

DIRECTIONS

1. In large pot or Dutch oven, heat olive oil over medium high heat.
2. Add pork cubes and cook, stirring occasionally for 4-6 minutes or until browned on all sides.
3. Add onion and garlic and cook for 2-3 minutes, or until starting to soften.
4. Add chipotle peppers and sauce, cumin, and seasoning packet. Stir to mix.
5. Add broth, tomatoes, beans and red pepper flakes if desired. Stir to mix well.
6. Bring stew to a boil then reduce heat to low.
7. Cover pot and simmer for 45 minutes to 1 hour, or until the port is fork tender.

8. Serve stew in bowls over brown rice or add rice to stew, if desired.

Asian Chicken Lettuce Wraps Recipe
INGREDIENTS
- 1 can (8 ounces) bamboo shoots, drained and minced
- 1 can (8 ounces) water chestnuts, drained and minced
- 3 tablespoons sherry cooking wine
- 2 tablespoons hoisin sauce
- 1 tablespoon unsalted peanut butter
- 2 teaspoons low-sodium soy sauce
- 2 teaspoons hot pepper sauce, such as Sriracha
- 2 packets (.035 ounce each) sugar substitute (such as Splenda)
- 1 tablespoon minced garlic
- 1 cup minced onion
- ½ pound ground chicken breast
- 1 teaspoon minced ginger
- ¼ teaspoon salt

- 1 teaspoon toasted sesame oil
- 8 small leaves butter lettuce
- 1 whole green onion, chopped
- 1 small cucumber, seeded and sliced into 1" strips

DIRECTIONS

1. In a medium bowl, combine the bamboo shoots, water chestnuts, sherry, hoisin sauce, peanut butter, soy sauce, hot-pepper sauce, and sugar substitute. Mix well. Set aside.
2. Mist a large, nonstick skillet with cooking spray and set over medium heat.
3. Add the onion and cook for 4 minutes or until onions are fragrant and softened.
4. Add the garlic and cook for a minute more.
5. Increase the heat to medium-high and add the ground chicken, ginger, and salt.
6. Cook, breaking up the chicken with a spatula or wooden spoon, for 3 to 4 minutes, until no longer pink.
7. Add the bamboo shoot and water chestnut mixture.

8. Cook for 2 minutes, or until heated through.
9. Stir in the toasted sesame oil.
10. Remove the pan from the heat.
11. To serve, divide the chicken mixture evening onto each of the 8 lettuce leaves.
12. Top with chopped green onion and cucumber. Serve immediately.

Chicken Cheesesteak Wrap Recipe
INGREDIENTS
- ¼ pound boneless, skinless chicken breast, trimmed of visible fat
- ¼ cup onions, chopped
- ¼ cup green pepper, sliced
- ¼ cup mushrooms, sliced
- 1 wedge (¾ ounce) Laughing Cow Original light swiss cheese or equivalent
- 1 whole wheat flour, low-carb tortilla
- 2 teaspoons sliced pickled hot chili peppers (optional)

DIRECTIONS

1. Place chicken breast on cutting board, pound to 1/4" thin and slice into very thin strips.
2. Place a skillet over medium high heat and mist with cooking spray.
3. Add the onion and chicken to the heated pan and cook until onions are translucent and chicken is no longer pink throughout.
4. Add green peppers and mushrooms to the pan and cook until peppers and mushrooms soften.
5. Place tortilla between 2 damp paper towels. Microwave for 20 seconds.
6. Lay the warm tortilla flat and spread cheese in an even strip in the middle.
7. Top with chicken, peppers, onions and mushrooms.
8. Add chili peppers if using.
9. Fold sides of tortilla over middle. Serve immediately.

Not Really Fried Rice Recipe
INGREDIENTS

- 2 tablespoons low-sodium soy sauce
- 1 teaspoon mustard
- 1 teaspoon chili paste
- 1 teaspoon toasted sesame oil
- 3 ounces boneless, skinless chicken breast cut into ½" cubes
- Black pepper, to taste
- ½ cup finely chopped whole green onions
- ¼ cup chopped carrot
- 1 clove garlic, minced
- ¾ cup cooked short-grain brown rice
- ¼ cup frozen peas
- 2 large egg whites
- Olive oil spray

DIRECTIONS

1. In a small bowl, combine soy sauce, mustard, chili paste and sesame oil. Set aside.
2. Season the cubed chicken with black pepper.
3. Mist a large, nonstick wok or skillet with cooking spray and place over medium high heat until it is hot enough for a drop of water to sizzle on it.

4. Scatter the chicken cubes into the wok or skillet.
5. Cook, stirring occasionally, until browned on all sides and no longer pink inside.
6. Transfer chicken to a plate and cover to keep warm.
7. Lightly mist the wok or skillet with cooking spray again. Set over medium-high heat.
8. Add the green onions, carrot, and garlic to the pan.
9. Cook, stirring frequently, for 2-3 minutes.
10. Add the cooked rice and peas.
11. Continue cooking and stirring for 2 minutes or until the mixture is hot throughout.
12. Using a spoon or spatula, create a hole in the rice and veggies to expose the center of the pan.
13. Off the heat, lightly mist the exposed part of the pan with cooking spray.
14. Add the egg whites and stir to mix them into the rice.

15. Cook for 1-2 minutes, or until the egg is completely cooked.
16. Return the chicken to the pan and stir in the reserved soy sauce mixture.
17. Leave on heat, stirring constantly, for about 1 minute or until heated. Serve immediately.

Egg-Chilada Recipe
INGREDIENTS
- 1 egg + 1 egg white
- Black pepper and salt to taste
- 1 ounce protein of choice (tofu, chicken, or ground beef work well)
- 2 tablespoons salsa (such as Tostito's medium)
- 1 tablespoon shredded Mexican blend cheese
- 2 tablespoons plain fat-free Greek yogurt

DIRECTIONS
1. Scramble the egg and egg white in a small bowl
2. Spray a skillet or griddle with cooking spray and set it over medium heat.

3. Pour the scrambled eggs onto the heated pan and allow it to spread into a generally circular shape.
4. Leave the eggs alone for a minute or two; allowing the edges to set. Add a sprinkle of black pepper and salt to the eggs while they're setting.
5. Slide a spatula beneath the eggs and flip (don't worry if some egg pours off at this point).
6. Cook eggs on the other side about two minutes or until completely cooked and transfer to a plate.
7. Make a strip of filling for your egg-chilada with 1 oz. protein of choice and Mexican cheese.
8. Roll up the egg "pancake" to form your egg-chilada.
9. Top with salsa and Greek yogurt.

Cheesecake Pudding Recipe
INGREDIENTS

- 1 cup plain fat-free Greek yogurt
- 1 package sugar-free cheesecake pudding mix

DIRECTIONS
1. Combine ingredients in a blender and puree until smooth.

Pan-Fried Rainbow Trout Recipe
INGREDIENTS
- 8 ounces rainbow trout fillets
- 3 Tbsp yellow cornmeal
- 1⅓ Tbsp chopped parsley
- ¼ tsp ground celery seeds
- ¼ tsp ground black pepper
- 1 pinch salt
- 2 tsp olive oil

DIRECTIONS
1. Clean and rinse fish fillets. Check to make sure all bones are removed. Pat dry.
2. Mix together cornmeal, salt, pepper, celery seed and chopped parsley.

3. Cover fish with cornmeal mixture and press onto fish.
4. Heat olive oil in non-stick skillet. Cook fish 2 to 3 minutes per side. Fish should be brown and crisp and should flake when pierced with a fork.

Pumpkin and Black Bean Soup Recipe
INGREDIENTS
- 2 tablespoons olive oil
- 1 medium onion, chopped
- 4 garlic cloves, minced
- 1 tablespoon ground cumin
- 1 teaspoon chili powder
- ½ teaspoon black pepper
- 2 cans (15 ounce) black beans, rinsed and drained
- 1 cup canned diced tomatoes
- 2 cups beef broth
- 1 can (16 ounce) pumpkin puree

DIRECTIONS

1. Heat oil in a soup kettle over medium heat, sauté onions, garlic, cumin, chili powder and pepper until soft.
2. Stir in black beans, tomatoes, broth and pumpkin.
3. Simmer uncovered stirring occasionally for about 25 minutes until soup is a thick consistency
4. Serve as is, or puree using an immersion blender for a smooth consistency.

SUGGESTIONS

Stir in plain Greek yogurt for added protein and creaminess.

Add ½-pound ground meat for an additional protein.

Asian Pork Tenderloin Recipe
INGREDIENTS
- ⅓ cup light soy sauce
- ⅓ cup brown sugar
- 2 tablespoons Worcestershire sauce
- 2 tablespoons lemon juice
- 2 tablespoons rice vinegar

- 1 tablespoon dry mustard
- 1 tablespoon ginger
- 1 ½ teaspoons pepper
- 4 garlic cloves or prepared minced
- 2 lbs pork tenderloin

DIRECTIONS
1. Mix ingredients together in freezer-safe bag.
2. Place tenderloin in freezer bag and rub marinade on pork.
3. Refrigerate overnight or place in freezer for future use.
4. Bake for 30-40 minutes at 375° F degrees OR prepare in slow cooker on low for 4-6 hours.

Greek Yogurt Chicken Recipe
INGREDIENTS
- 4 boneless skinless chicken breasts (4 ounces each)
- 1 cup plain Greek yogurt
- ½ cup grated Parmesan cheese
- 1 teaspoon garlic powder
- 1 ½ teaspoons seasoning salt

- ½ teaspoon pepper

DIRECTIONS

1. Preheat oven to 375 degrees.
2. Combine Greek yogurt, cheese and seasonings in bowl.
3. Line baking sheet with foil and spray with cooking spray.
4. Coat each chicken breast in Greek yogurt mixture and place on foiled baking sheet.
5. Bake for 45 minutes.
6. Enjoy!!

High-Protein Cottage Cheese Pancakes Recipe
INGREDIENTS

- ⅓ cup all-purpose flour
- ½ tsp baking soda
- 1 cup low-fat cottage cheese
- ½ tablespoons canola oil
- 3 eggs, lightly beaten

DIRECTIONS

1. Combine flour and baking soda in a small bowl.

2. Combine remaining ingredients in a large bowl.
3. Pour flour mixture into cottage cheese mixture and stir until just incorporated.
4. Heat a large skillet over medium heat, coat with cooking spray.
5. Pour ? cup portions of batter onto skillet and cook until bubbles appear on the surface.
6. Flip and cook on the other side until brown.
7. Serve with low calorie syrup.

Spicy Deviled Eggs Recipe

INGREDIENTS

- 6 hard-boiled eggs (You will not use three of the yolks in this recipe.)
- 2 Tablespoons of creamy horseradish sauce or Greek yogurt
- ½ teaspoon dill
- ¼ teaspoon spicy mustard (Use Dijon for mild deviled eggs.)
- ⅛ teaspoon salt
- Dash of black pepper and paprika

DIRECTIONS

1. Peel the eggs and cut in half lengthwise.
2. Place 3 yolks into a mixing bowl, and set the whites aside. (Save the other three yolks for another use.)
3. Mash the yolks with creamy horseradish sauce or Greek yogurt, dill, mustard and salt.
4. Spoon or pipe filling into egg white halves.
5. Sprinkle with pepper and paprika.

Slow-Cooker Chicken Taco Filling Recipe
INGREDIENTS
- 16 ounce (1 lb) skinless, boneless chicken breasts
- 1 cup chicken broth
- 1 (1.25 ounce) package dry taco seasoning mix

INSTRUCTIONS
1. Mix chicken broth and taco seasoning in a bowl.
2. Place chicken breast in slow cooker.
3. Pour broth and seasoning mixture over chicken.

4. Cover and cook on low for 6-8 hours.
5. Shred chicken.
6. Cook on low for additional 30 minutes to absorb excess juices.
7. Serve as filling for tacos, topping for a salad or by itself for a protein source.

Thai Tofu Quinoa Bowl Recipe
INGREDIENTS
- 1 package extra firm tofu (15 oz), diced
- 2 tablespoons soy sauce
- 1 tablespoon sesame oil
- 1 cup uncooked quinoa
- 1½ cups chicken broth
- ½ cup slivered almonds
- 1 cup shredded carrots
- 2/3 cup chopped scallions
- ½ cup fresh cilantro

For the sauce:
- 2 teaspoons creamy peanut butter
- 2 tablespoons Sriracha sauce
- 2 tablespoons rice wine vinegar

- 3 tablespoons coconut milk
- ½ tablespoon brown sugar
- 1 garlic clove, minced
- ½ lime, juiced
- 1 teaspoon grated ginger

INSTRUCTIONS

1. 30 minutes before cooking, drain and rinse tofu.
   - Wrap in clean dish towel and place on rimmed dinner plate.
   - Place another plate on top and weight down with something heavy to press out some of the excess liquid.
   - Let sit 15-30 minutes.
2. Preheat oven to 350? F.
3. Toss tofu, soy sauce and sesame oil in bowl.
4. Place tofu in single layer on lined baking sheet.
5. Bake for 35-40 minutes tossing every ten minutes to crisp tofu on all sides.
6. Toast and cook quinoa.
   - Place a medium sizes sauce pan on medium low heat.

- Add in dry quinoa and toast for 5 minutes, stirring occasionally until golden brown.
- Add broth to quinoa, lower heat slightly.
- Cover and cook for 12-15 minutes or until all liquid is absorbed.
- Fluff with a fork and set aside.

7. Make the sauce:
   - Place peanut butter in bowl and microwave for 10 seconds to melt.
   - Add remaining ingredients and whisk well to combine.
8. Toast the almonds:
   - Place almonds in small sauce pan.
   - Cook on medium low heat, stirring occasionally until almonds are golden grown.
9. Toss together quinoa, vegetables, herbs, tofu, and nuts.
10. Pour sauce over everything and toss to combine. ENJOY!

Baked Tomatoes Recipe
INGREDIENTS

- 5-6 large tomatoes
- Olive oil spray
- ¼ cup low fat parmesan cheese
- Greek Seasoning (Penzey's is preferred)
- ¼ cup pine nuts (optional)

INSTRUCTIONS
1. Preheat oven to 350° F.
2. Cut tomatoes in half-lengthwise and place open face in non-stick 9x13 pan.
3. Spray surface of tomatoes with olive oil spray.
4. Coat with cheese and pine nuts.
5. Sprinkle on Greek seasoning to taste.
6. Bake for 50 minutes on middle rack.

Slow-Cooker Chicken Tikka Masala Recipe
INGREDIENTS
- 3 lbs boneless, skinless chicken breast
- 1 large onion, diced
- 4 cloves garlic, minced
- 2 tbsp fresh ginger, minced
- 1 can tomato puree (29 oz)

- 1½ cups plain Greek yogurt (12 oz)
- 2 tbsp olive oil
- 2 tbsp Garam masala
- 1 tbsp cumin
- ½ tbsp paprika
- ¾ tsp cinnamon
- ¾ tsp ground black pepper
- 1-3 tsp cayenne pepper (depending on taste)
- 2 bay leaves
- Chopped cilantro for topping

INSTRUCTIONS

1. Place everything up to bay leaves in large bowl.
2. With a spatula, stir to combine and coat chicken well.
3. Gently place into slow cooker, add bay leaves on top.
4. Cover and cook for 8 hours on low or 4 hours on high.
5. Remove bay leaves, and serve topped with cilantro.

Ginger Beef Stir Fry Recipe
INGREDIENTS
- 1 pound flank steak (cut into ¼-inch strips)
- 2 teaspoons ground ginger
- 2 medium garlic cloves
- 6 ounces beef broth (fat free)
- ¼ cup (2 ounces) hoisin sauce
- 3 tablespoons soy sauce
- 1 tablespoons cornstarch
- 1 teaspoon canola oil
- ¼ teaspoon crushed red pepper flakes
- 3 ounces broccoli florets
- ½ medium yellow, red or green bell pepper cut into strips
- ½ cup instant brown rice
- 2 medium stalks bok choy cut into ½-inch slices
- 8-ounce can sliced water chestnuts

INSTRUCTIONS
1. In mixing bowl, stir together steak, garlic and ginger. Set aside.

2. Prepare rice according to directions on package.
3. Combine broth, hoisin sauce, soy sauce and cornstarch in a bowl. Stir until dissolved.
4. In wok or skillet, heat oil and red pepper flakes over medium-high heat.
5. Cook steak 4-5 minutes or until browned. Stir constantly. Set aside.
6. Put broccoli, bell pepper and carrot into pan. Cook over medium-high heat for 2-3 minutes or until tender-crisp. Stir. (If mixture becomes too dry, add in 1-2 tablespoons water.)
7. Stir in bok choy and water chestnuts. Cook for additional 1-2 minutes or under bok choy is tender-crisp. Stir constantly.
8. Make a well in center of pan, and pour in broth.
9. Cook 1-2 minutes or until broth thickens, occasionally stir broth.
10. Mix in beef. Cook 1-2 minutes or until warm.
11. Serve over rice.

Classic Hummus Recipe

INGREDIENTS
- 1 clove garlic, smashed and peeled
- 1 15-ounce can chickpeas, rinsed
- 3 tablespoons fresh lemon juice
- 3 tablespoons extra-virgin olive oil
- 1 tablespoon tahini
- ½ teaspoon salt

INSTRUCTIONS
1. In food processor, chop garlic until finely minced.
2. Scrape down the sides of food processor and add chickpeas, lemon juice, oil, tahini, and salt.
3. Process until completely smooth, scraping down sides as necessary (1-2 minutes).

Cajun Chicken Stuffed With Pepper Jack Cheese and Spinach Recipe

INGREDIENTS
- 1 lb (16 oz) boneless, skinless chicken breasts

- 3 oz reduced fat pepper jack cheese (Shredded)
- 1 cup frozen spinach thawed and drained (or fresh cooked)
- 2 tsp olive oil
- 2 tbsp Cajun seasoning (see recipe below if you want to make homemade)
- 1 tbsp bread crumbs
- Toothpicks

INSTRUCTIONS

1. Preheat oven to 350° F degrees.
2. Flatten the chicken to 1/4-inch thickness.
3. In a medium bowl, combine the pepper jack cheese, spinach, salt and pepper.
4. Combine the Cajun seasoning and breadcrumbs together in a small bowl.
5. Spoon about 1/4 c of the spinach mixture onto each chicken breast. Roll each chicken breast tightly and fasten the seams with several toothpicks.

6. Brush each chicken breast with the olive oil. Sprinkle the Cajun seasoning mixture evenly over all.
7. Sprinkle any remaining spinach and cheese on top of chicken (optional).
8. Place the chicken seam-side up onto a tin foil-lined baking sheet (for easy cleanup).
9. Bake for 35 to 40 minutes, or until chicken is cooked through.
10. Remove the toothpicks before serving. Count to make sure you have removed every last toothpick.
11. Serve whole or slice into medallions.

Cajun Seasoning (makes approximately 2 tablespoons)
- ¾ tbsp paprika
- ¾ tsp onion powder
- ¾ tsp garlic powder
- ¼ tsp black pepper
- ½ tsp cayenne pepper
- ¼ tsp white pepper
- ¼ tsp cumin

- ¼ tsp thyme
- ¼ tsp oregano

Chicken Rollantini with Spinach ala Parmigiana Recipe

INGREDIENTS

- 8 chicken breast cutlets (pounded thin)—3 oz each
- ½ cup whole wheat Italian seasoned breadcrumbs
- ¼ cup grated parmesan cheese, divided
- 6 tablespoons egg whites/egg beaters, divided
- 5 oz frozen spinach, thawed and squeezed dry of any liquid
- 6 tbsp part skim ricotta cheese
- 6 oz part skim mozzarella—shredded, divided
- Non-stick cooking spray
- 1 cup marinara sauce

INSTRUCTIONS

1. Preheat oven to 450° degrees

2. Spray 9x13 glass baking dish with non-stick cooking spray.
3. Season chicken cutlets with salt & pepper
4. In a small bowl, combine breadcrumbs with 2 tablespoons grated parmesan cheese.
5. Place ¼ cup egg whites in another bowl.
6. Combine 1.5 oz mozzarella cheese with remaining grated parmesan cheese, spinach, remaining 2 tbsp egg whites, and ricotta cheese.
7. Lay seasoned, pounded chicken cutlets on working surface and spread 2 tbsp of spinach-cheese mixtures on each.
8. Loosely roll each cutlet, keeping the seam side down and secure with a toothpick or two.
9. Dip the chicken rolls in egg whites, then in breadcrumb mixture and place seam-side down in greased baking dish.
10. Repeat with remaining chicken.
11. Lightly spray chicken rollantinis with non-stick spray.

12. Bake 25 minutes, or until instant-read thermometer reads 165°F.
13. Remove, top with marinara sauce and remaining shredded mozzarella cheese.
14. Bake for 3 more minutes, until cheese is melted and bubbling.
15. Serve with additional sauce on side and grated parmesan cheese.

Cottage Cheese Fluff Recipe

INGREDIENTS

- 2 24-ounce containers fat-free cottage cheese
- 1 8-ounce sugar-free whipped topping
- 2 0.3-ounce packages sugar-free gelatin, flavor of choice

DIRECTIONS

1. Mix all ingredients in a large bowl.
2. Optional — add your favorite fruit.

Zucchini Boat Recipe

INGREDIENTS

- 4 medium zucchini

- 1 pound ground turkey breast
- ½ cup chopped onion
- 1 egg, beaten
- ½ lbs sliced mushrooms
- 1 large tomato diced
- ¾ cup spaghetti sauce
- ¼ cup seasoned whole wheat bread crumbs
- ¼ teaspoon salt
- ¼ teaspoon pepper
- 1 cup (4 ounces) shredded low fat mozzarella cheese

DIRECTIONS

1. Cut zucchini in half lengthwise; cut a thin slice from the bottom of each with a sharp knife to allow zucchini to sit flat.
2. Scoop out pulp, leaving ¼-in. shells. Set pulp aside.
3. Place shells in an ungreased 3-qt. microwave-safe dish. Cover and microwave on high for 3 minutes or until crisp-tender; drain and set aside.

4. In a large skillet, cook ground turkey and onion over medium heat until meat is no longer pink; drain. Remove from the heat.
5. In a large bowl mix together zucchini pulp, beaten egg, spaghetti sauce, bread crumbs, mushrooms, tomato, salt, pepper, ½ cup cheese and cooked ground turkey.
6. Spoon about ¼ cup mixture into each shell.
7. Sprinkle with remaining cheese.
8. Bake uncovered for 20 minutes at 350° F or until brown.

Egg Muffin Recipe
INGREDIENTS
- 6 large eggs
- 12 slices pre-cooked turkey bacon (sliced into thirds)
- ¾ cup shredded low fat Swiss or Monterey jack cheese
- ½ cup 1% milk
- ¼ teaspoon salt
- ¼ teaspoon pepper

- ¼ teaspoon Italian seasoning

DIRECTIONS
1. Spray muffin tin with nonstick cooking spray.
2. Preheat oven to 350° F.
3. Place 3 bacon pieces in the bottom of each muffin cup.
4. In a separate bowl, mix together all ingredients until well blended, except for ¼ cup of the shredded cheese.
5. Fill each muffin cup with ¼ cup of the egg mixture.
6. Sprinkle extra ¼ cup of cheese on top across muffins.
7. Bake for 20-25 minutes or until eggs are set.

Cottage Cheese Bake Recipe
INGREDIENTS
- 2 cups low-fat or fat-free cottage cheese
- 2 whole eggs
- 10-ounce pack of frozen spinach (thawed and drained)

- ½ cup Parmesan cheese

DIRECTIONS
1. Preheat oven to 350° F.
2. In large bowl, mix all ingredients together well.
3. Place evenly into 8x8 pan.
4. Bake for 20-30 minutes or until cheese bubbles on outside.
5. Let sit 5 minutes before serving.
6. Season to taste with salt, pepper, and garlic as desired.

Tofu and Broccoli Quiche Recipe
INGREDIENTS
- ½ cup uncooked bulgur wheat
- Pinch of salt
- 1 tablespoon sesame oil
- 1 yellow onion, chopped
- ½ pound broccoli, chopped
- ¼ pound mushrooms, chopped
- 1½ pounds tofu
- 2 tablespoons sesame tahini

- 1 tablespoon umeboshi paste (pickled plum paste) or white miso
- 1 tablespoon tamari

DIRECTIONS

1. Preheat oven to 350?F.
2. Bring 1 cup water to a boil in a small pot, add bulgur and salt and return to a boil.
3. Lower heat, cover and cook for 15 minutes.
4. Press hot bulgur into a greased 9-inch pie pan and baked for 12 minutes, or until somewhat dry and crust-like. Set aside.
5. Heat oil in a large skillet over medium high heat.
6. Add onions, broccoli and mushrooms to skillet and cook briefly.
7. Cover skillet and turn off heat; set aside while you prepare tofu mixture.
8. Blend tofu, tahini, umeboshi paste and tamari in a food processor until smooth.
9. Transfer mixture to a bowl and add cooked vegetables. Toss gently to combine.

10. Pour vegetable mixture into bulgur crust, then bake for 30 minutes.
11. Remove from oven and let sit for 10 minutes.
12. Cut into 6 slices slices and serve hot or cold.

Faux Fried Chicken Recipe
INGREDIENTS
- ⅓ cup reduced-fat buttermilk
- ⅛ tsp. paprika
- 12 oz. raw boneless skinless lean chicken breast tenders (about 10 pieces)
- ⅓ cup bran cereal (Original Fiber One® or similar type)
- ⅓ cup panko breadcrumbs
- 1 Tbsp. dry onion soup mix
- Optional: salt, to taste

DIRECTIONS
1. In a large sealable container or plastic bag, combine buttermilk with paprika and mix well.
2. Add chicken and coat completely. Seal and refrigerate for at least 1 hour.

3. Preheat oven to 375 degrees.
4. Prepare a large baking sheet by spraying it with nonstick spray. Set aside.
5. Using a blender or food processor, grind cereal to a breadcrumb-like consistency. Pour crumbs into a large bowl.
6. Add panko breadcrumbs and onion soup mix. If you like, add a dash or two of salt. Mix thoroughly.
7. One at a time, remove each piece of chicken from container/bag, give it a shake (to get rid of excess buttermilk), coat it evenly with the crumb mixture, and lay it flat on the baking sheet.
8. Bake in the oven for 10 minutes. Flip carefully (tongs work well!), and then bake for an additional 10 minutes, or until outsides are crispy and chicken is cooked through.

Cheesy Vegetarian Chili Recipe
INGREDIENTS
- 2 garlic cloves

- 2 teaspoons olive oil
- 1 large green bell pepper (diced)
- 1 cup onion chopped
- ½ pound of sliced mushrooms
- 14.5-ounce can of diced tomatoes or 2 cups fresh tomatoes
- 8 ounces tomato sauce
- 2 tablespoons chili powder
- 1 medium zucchini (thinly sliced)
- 2 15-ounce cans red kidney beans (rinsed)
- 10-ounce package of frozen corn
- 1 cup low fat shredded cheddar cheese

DIRECTIONS

1. Heat olive oil and garlic in large pan.
2. Add onions, green pepper, and mushrooms. Cook until tender.
3. Add in tomato sauce, diced tomatoes, chili powder, and bring to boil.
4. Turn down to low, add in zucchini and kidney beans. Simmer for 10-15 minutes.
5. Add frozen corn and ½ cup cheddar cheese. Stir.
6. Simmer on low for additional 10-15 minutes.
7. Serve topped with cheddar cheese.

Creamy Slow Cooker Chicken Recipe
INGREDIENTS

- 6 skinless, boneless chicken breasts (2½ lb.)
- 10¾ ounce reduced fat cream of mushroom soup
- 1 cup pureed cottage cheese or plain Greek yogurt
- ½ cup chicken stock
- 0.7 ounce envelope Italian dressing mix

- 8 ounce pkg mushrooms
- Cooking spray

DIRECTIONS

1. Spray a large skillet with cooking spray. Cook chicken in batches over medium-high heat 2-3 minutes on each side or until just browned. Transfer chicken to a 5-qt. slow cooker.
2. Add soup, cottage cheese or yogurt, chicken stock, and Italian dressing mix to skillet. Cook over medium heat, stirring constantly, 2 to 3 minutes or until cheese is melted and mixture is smooth.
3. Arrange mushrooms over chicken in slow cooker. Spoon soup mixture over mushrooms. Cover and cook on LOW 4 hours. Stir well before serving.
4. To make ahead: Prepare recipe as directed. Transfer to a 13- x 9-inch baking dish, and let cool completely. Freeze up to one month. Thaw in refrigerator 8 to 24 hours. To reheat, cover tightly with aluminum foil, and bake at

325? for 45 minutes. Uncover and bake 15 minutes or until thoroughly heated.

Cheesy Crustless Quiche Recipe
INGREDIENTS
- 4 ounces cubed baby low fat Swiss
- 6 ounces grilled chicken breast, cut up into 1" cubes
- 10 ounces shredded low fat mozzarella cheese
- 3 large eggs
- 1 cup skim milk
- Oregano to season (if desired)
- Nonstick cooking spray
- 9" pie pan

DIRECTIONS
1. Preheat oven to 400 degrees.
2. Spray pie pan with non-stick cooking spray.
3. Fill the pie pan with the cubed baby Swiss and cubed chicken breast.
4. Spread the 2 cups of shredded mozzarella cheese over the top of the entire mixture.

5. Sprinkle the oregano on the top to taste.
6. In a separate bowl, whip together the eggs and skim milk. Pour over the chicken and cheese.
7. Bake at 400 degrees for 40 minutes. (The top will be very lightly browned when finished.)
8. Let cool and serve immediately or cover with tinfoil and place in refrigerator.
1. Feel free to add cooked vegetables to preferences — tomatoes, onions, green pepper.

Cheesy Stuffed Acorn Squash Recipe
INGREDIENTS
- 2 acorn squash, halved and seeded
- 1 lbs (16 oz) extra lean ground turkey breast
- 1 cup diced celery
- 1 cup finely chopped onion
- 1 cup fresh mushrooms, sliced
- 1 teaspoon basil
- 1 teaspoon oregano
- 1 teaspoon garlic powder

- 1/8 teaspoon salt
- 1 pinch ground black pepper
- 8 oz can tomato sauce
- 1 cup reduced fat shredded Cheddar cheese

DIRECTIONS

1. Preheat oven to 350 degrees F (175 degrees C).
2. Place squash cut side down in a glass dish.
3. Cook in microwave for 20 minutes on HIGH, until almost tender.
4. In a non-stick saucepan over medium heat, brown ground turkey.
5. Add celery and onion; sauté until transparent.
6. Stir in mushrooms; cook 2 to 3 minutes more.
7. Add in tomato sauce and dry seasonings
8. Divide mixture into quarters, spoon into the squash and cover.
9. Cook 15 minutes in the preheated 350 degrees F (175 degrees C) oven.
10. Uncover, sprinkle with cheese and put back in the oven until the cheese bubbles.

CONCLUSION

The pre-op diet largely consists of protein shakes and other high-protein, low-calorie foods that are easy to digest. Protein helps bolster and protect muscle tissue. This can help your body burn fat instead of muscle for fuel. Protein also helps keep your body strong, which can speed up recovery.

As the date for your surgery nears, you may need to follow a mostly-liquid or liquid-only diet. Based on your weight and overall health, your doctor may allow you to eat some solids during this time. These might include fish, watered-down hot cereal, or soft-boiled eggs.

Before the surgery, make sure you ask the anesthesiologist for instructions about what you can or can't have before the surgery. These suggestions may vary depending on your situation. For example, your doctor may want you to drink carbohydrate-rich fluids up to 2 hours before surgery.

For the first four weeks following a gastric bypass operation you will need to follow a liquid diet menu.

A liquid diet consists of pureed, smooth and lump free foods.

Eating only liquid diet food for four weeks can get a little boring and therefore it is a good idea to prepare your meals well in advance before your gastric bypass procedure.

This is particularly important if you have little support in the home and usually prepare your own food as preparing your liquid diet food could be challenging while recovering from a major operation.

Remember to eat slowly and chew each bite very slowly and completely. DO NOT swallow food until it is smooth. The opening between your new stomach pouch and your intestines is very small. Food that is not chewed well can block this opening.

Some foods you eat may cause some pain or discomfort if you do not chew them completely. Some of these are pasta, rice, bread, raw vegetables, and meats. Adding a low-fat sauce, broth, or gravy can make them easier to digest. Other foods that may cause discomfort are dry foods, such as popcorn and nuts, or fibrous foods, such as celery and corn.

Made in United States
Orlando, FL
13 July 2023